Published by Jehu Press AUSTRALIA
Illustrations by Freekpik.com

Overview of the Book: Fit in Fifteen Plan: Fitness for Busy People (Coach's Perspective)

Welcome to the Fit in Fifteen Plan: Fitness for Busy People! As a coach, I'm excited to introduce you to this comprehensive guide that will help you achieve your fitness goals despite a busy lifestyle. This book is designed to provide you with practical strategies, effective workouts, and nutritional guidance to help you prioritize your health and fitness, even when time is limited.

The Fit in Fifteen Plan is rooted in the belief that everyone deserves the opportunity to lead a healthy and active life, regardless of their schedule. This book is not about spending hours in the gym or following restrictive diets. Instead, it focuses on optimizing your fitness journey by maximizing your workout time and making mindful nutrition choices in just fifteen minutes at a time.

Throughout the book, you'll find a step-by-step approach to building a sustainable fitness routine that fits seamlessly into your busy lifestyle. You'll learn how to leverage high-intensity workouts, including cardiovascular exercises and strength training, to achieve maximum results in minimal time. We'll explore the principles of High-Intensity Interval Training (HIIT) and provide you with sample workout routines that can be completed in just fifteen minutes, four days a week.

Nutrition plays a crucial role in achieving your fitness goals, and we'll guide you through making smart food choices and practicing portion control, even when time is limited. You'll discover quick and nutritious meal ideas that can be prepared and enjoyed within your fifteen-minute windows.

In addition to the workout and nutrition guidance, we'll delve into essential topics such as goal setting, assessing your fitness level, creating a supportive environment, and maintaining long-term success. We'll provide strategies for managing your time effectively, incorporating fitness into your daily activities, and developing a growth mindset that will propel you forward on your fitness journey.

As your coach, my goal is to empower you to take control of your health and well-being, despite the demands of a busy life. Whether you're a working professional, a busy parent, or someone juggling multiple responsibilities, this book will provide you with the tools, knowledge, and support to prioritize your fitness goals and achieve lasting success.

Remember, fitness is not an all-or-nothing endeavor. Small, consistent efforts can lead to significant results. By dedicating just fifteen minutes, four days a week, and making mindful nutrition choices, you can transform your health and fitness. Together, we'll navigate the challenges of a busy lifestyle and unlock your full potential.

Let's embark on this journey together, embrace the Fit in Fifteen Plan, and create a healthier, fitter, and more energized version of yourself. Get ready to make fitness a non-negotiable part of your busy life!

Disclaimer:

Before starting any fitness program, it is important to consult with a qualified healthcare professional, such as your doctor or a certified fitness trainer. The information provided in the "Fit in Fifteen Plan: Fitness for Busy People" eBook is for educational purposes only and should not be considered a substitute for professional medical advice, diagnosis, or treatment.

1. Consultation with a Healthcare Professional:

- It is essential to consult with your doctor or healthcare professional before beginning any new fitness program, especially if you have any pre-existing medical conditions or injuries.

- Your healthcare provider can assess your overall health and advise you on the suitability of the Fit in Fifteen Plan based on your specific circumstances.

2. Pregnancy and Postpartum:

- If you are pregnant or postpartum, it is crucial to consult with your obstetrician or healthcare provider before starting any exercise program.

- Certain exercises may not be suitable or safe during pregnancy or postpartum recovery, and it is important to receive professional guidance tailored to your individual situation.

3. Individualized Modifications:

- The Fit in Fifteen Plan provides general fitness guidelines and recommendations. However, everyone's fitness level and abilities are unique.

- It is important to listen to your body and make appropriate modifications to exercises to ensure your safety and prevent injury.

- If you have any concerns or questions about specific exercises or movements, consult with a certified fitness professional for personalized guidance.

4. Risk of Injury:

- Participating in physical exercise carries inherent risks of injury.

- It is essential to perform exercises with proper form, technique, and appropriate intensity to minimize the risk of injury.

- If you experience any pain, discomfort, or dizziness during exercise, stop immediately and consult with a healthcare professional.

5. Individual Responsiblity:

- Every individual is responsible for their own health and well-being.

- By engaging in the Fit in Fifteen Plan, you acknowledge that you are participating voluntarily and assume all risks associated with the program.

- It is important to use common sense, listen to your body, and make informed decisions regarding your fitness activities.

Remember, the Fit in Fifteen Plan is designed to provide general fitness information and guidance. It is not intended to replace professional medical advice. Always consult with your healthcare provider before starting any new exercise or fitness program, particularly if you have any underlying health concerns or are pregnant or postpartum. Your healthcare professional can provide personalized recommendations based on your individual needs and circumstances.

Table of Contents:

Chapter 1: Introduction

The "Fit in Fifteen Plan: Fitness for Busy People" eBook is a comprehensive resource designed to help individuals with packed schedules prioritize their fitness goals. This practical guide offers a time-efficient approach to exercise and nutrition, allowing busy individuals to achieve significant results without compromising their limited time.

The eBook presents a strategic four-day-per-week workout plan that combines high-intensity weight training and cardio exercises. These intense 15-minute workouts are carefully crafted to maximize efficiency and deliver effective fitness outcomes. Whether you are a beginner or an experienced fitness enthusiast, the exercises provided can be tailored to your fitness level, ensuring a challenging yet manageable routine.

Recognizing the significance of rest and recovery, the Fit in Fifteen Plan also incorporates three dedicated rest days. These rest periods allow your body to heal and rebuild, reducing the risk of injury and enabling you to perform at your best during workouts.

In addition to the workout component, the eBook emphasizes the importance of a well-balanced diet. It introduces the concept of organizing 15-minute windows for meals, providing structure and guidance for maintaining a consistent and nourishing eating routine. While the meals may be shorter in duration, the focus is on selecting nutrient-dense foods that fuel your body and support your fitness goals.

The Fit in Fifteen Plan is specifically designed for individuals leading busy lives, such as professionals, parents, or individuals constantly on the go. By dedicating just a fraction of your day to exercise and mindful eating, you can improve your overall health, boost your energy levels, and achieve the fit and active lifestyle you desire.

Take the first step towards a healthier and fitter you by exploring the "Fit in Fifteen Plan: Fitness for Busy People" eBook. Discover a time-efficient approach to fitness that seamlessly integrates into your busy lifestyle and empowers you to make lasting positive changes.

Chapter 2: Understanding the Fit in Fifteen Philosophy

In Chapter 2 of the "Fit in Fifteen Plan: Fitness for Busy People" eBook, we delve into the core principles and philosophy behind this time-efficient approach to fitness. By understanding the concepts outlined in this chapter, you will gain valuable insights into the effectiveness and benefits of the Fit in Fifteen Plan for your busy lifestyle.

The Fit in Fifteen Philosophy revolves around maximizing your time and effort to achieve significant results. It recognizes the constraints faced by busy individuals and offers practical solutions to overcome these challenges while still prioritizing health and fitness.

One of the key aspects of this philosophy is the concept of time efficiency. Traditional workouts often require long durations, making it difficult for busy individuals to consistently fit them into their schedules. The Fit in Fifteen Plan challenges this notion by emphasizing shorter, focused workouts that can be completed in just 15 minutes. We believe that these intense bursts of exercise, when done correctly, can yield remarkable results in a fraction of the time.

High-intensity training lies at the heart of the Fit in Fifteen Philosophy. This chapter explores the science behind high-intensity workouts and their impact on fitness and overall health. By engaging in intense bursts of exercise, you can stimulate your cardiovascular system, enhance muscle strength and endurance, and boost your metabolism. We delve into the physiological benefits of these workouts, including improved cardiovascular fitness, increased calorie burn, and the release of endorphins that contribute to an elevated mood.

While high-intensity workouts offer numerous benefits, it's crucial to strike a balance between intensity and safety. This chapter provides insights into finding the appropriate level of challenge while ensuring proper form and technique. We offer guidelines on gradually increasing intensity, listening to your body's signals, and knowing when to modify exercises to prevent injury and promote long-term success.

Finally, we address the common obstacles and excuses that often prevent individuals from prioritizing fitness. By acknowledging these challenges, we can develop strategies to overcome them. This chapter provides practical tips and techniques to overcome time constraints, combat fatigue, and create a mindset of commitment to your health and well-being.

Understanding the Fit in Fifteen Philosophy is essential as it forms the foundation for the subsequent chapters, where we'll guide you through the specifics of the Fit in Fifteen Plan, including workouts, nutrition, and strategies for incorporating fitness into your busy lifestyle.

Prepare to embark on a fitness journey that leverages the power of time efficiency and empowers you to achieve optimal results in just 15 minutes a day. The Fit in Fifteen Philosophy will revolutionize your approach to fitness and help you unlock your full potential while navigating your busy life.

Chapter 3: Setting Your Fitness Goals

In Chapter 3 of the "Fit in Fifteen Plan: Fitness for Busy People" eBook, we dive into the crucial step of setting your fitness goals. Understanding the importance of goal setting and creating a clear vision for your fitness journey is essential to stay motivated and track your progress effectively. In this chapter, we will guide you through the process of setting meaningful and achievable fitness goals, providing you with the knowledge and tools to turn your aspirations into reality.

1. The Significance of Goal Setting

Setting specific, measurable, attainable, relevant, and time-bound (SMART) goals is crucial for your fitness journey. By establishing clear objectives, you provide yourself with direction and purpose. Goals serve as a roadmap, helping you stay focused and motivated throughout your fitness journey. Additionally, achieving your goals provides a sense of accomplishment and boosts your confidence, reinforcing your commitment to a healthy lifestyle.

2. Assessing Your Current Fitness Level

Before setting your goals, it's important to assess your current fitness level. This assessment serves as a baseline for measuring your progress and helps you identify areas that require improvement. Evaluate your strength, endurance, flexibility, and cardiovascular fitness through various fitness tests or consultations with a fitness professional. Understanding where you stand allows you to set realistic and appropriate goals tailored to your starting point.

3. Defining Your Fitness Objectives

Fitness goals vary from person to person based on individual desires and aspirations. Identify the specific areas of fitness you wish to improve, whether it's weight loss, muscle gain, cardiovascular endurance, or overall health improvement. These goals should align with your personal values and provide intrinsic motivation. Take the time to reflect on what truly matters to you and craft objectives that resonate with your aspirations.

4. Creating Actionable Goals

Transforming your fitness objectives into actionable goals is essential for progress. Break down your overarching goals into smaller, manageable steps that you can easily track and achieve. By setting both short-term and long-term goals, you create a series of milestones that celebrate your progress along the way. Each milestone acts as a building block towards your ultimate objective, keeping you motivated and engaged.

5. Tracking Progress and Staying Accountable

Tracking your progress is essential to monitor your advancements and stay accountable to your goals. Explore various methods of tracking, such as keeping a workout journal, utilizing fitness apps, or wearing wearable devices. Regularly assess and record key metrics like body measurements, weight, and fitness performance to objectively measure your progress. Additionally, consider sharing your goals with a supportive community or finding an accountability partner who can provide encouragement, guidance, and support throughout your journey.

6. Adjusting and Reevaluating Goals

As you progress on your fitness journey, goals may need to be adjusted or modified to align with your changing needs, preferences, and capabilities. Regularly reevaluate your goals to ensure they remain relevant and challenging. Adapt your goals based on your evolving fitness level and lifestyle circumstances, while still maintaining the intrinsic motivation that drove you to set them initially.

By setting clear and meaningful fitness goals, you empower yourself to take charge of your health and well-being. The Fit in Fifteen Plan provides the framework, guidance, and support to help you achieve your aspirations. Embrace the opportunity to define your fitness goals, and let the Fit in Fifteen Plan be your companion as you embark on an exciting journey towards a healthier and fitter you. Remember, with dedication and a well-defined vision, you can turn your dreams into achievable milestones and celebrate the transformative power of fitness.

Chapter 4: The Fit in Fifteen Workout Framework

Welcome to Chapter 4 of the "Fit in Fifteen Plan: Fitness for Busy People" eBook! In this chapter, I'm going to walk you through the Fit in Fifteen Workout Framework, just like a personal trainer would. This framework is designed to help you make the most of your 15-minute workout sessions, ensuring that you get a challenging and effective workout within a limited timeframe. So, let's get started!

1. Warm-Up and Mobility:

- Before diving into your workout, it's crucial to warm up your muscles and increase your joint mobility.

- Start with 5-10 minutes of light cardio, such as jogging in place, jumping jacks, or brisk walking.

- Follow it up with dynamic stretches and mobility exercises to loosen up your muscles and prepare them for the upcoming workout.

- Incorporate movements like arm circles, leg swings, hip rotations, and shoulder rolls to target major muscle groups.

2. High-Intensity Interval Training (HIIT):

- HIIT is a fantastic way to maximize your workout in a short amount of time.

- Choose 2-3 exercises that target different muscle groups and get your heart rate up.

- Perform each exercise for 30 seconds to 1 minute with maximum effort, followed by 15-30 seconds of rest.

- Repeat this cycle for a total of 3-4 sets.

- Examples of HIIT exercises include burpees, mountain climbers, squat jumps, high knees, or jumping lunges.

- You can mix and match exercises based on your fitness level and equipment availability.

3. Weight Training:

- Weight training is essential for building strength, toning muscles, and boosting metabolism.

- Choose compound exercises that work multiple muscle groups simultaneously, allowing you to get the most out of your workout.

- Select weights that challenge you but still allow you to maintain proper form and technique.

- Perform 2-3 sets of 8-12 repetitions for each exercise, resting for 30-60 seconds between sets.

- Some examples of weight training exercises include squats, lunges, push-ups, shoulder presses, or bicep curls.

4. Cardiovascular Conditioning:

- Cardiovascular exercises are crucial for improving your heart health, stamina, and calorie burn.

- Incorporate cardio exercises that get your heart rate up and engage large muscle groups.

- Aim for 5-10 minutes of continuous cardio, such as jogging in place, jumping rope, high knees, or cycling.

- Adjust the intensity and speed based on your fitness level and available space or equipment.

5. Cool-Down and Stretching:

- After completing your workout, it's important to cool down your body and stretch your muscles to prevent tightness and promote recovery.

- Slow down the intensity of your movements and perform 5-10 minutes of light cardio, such as walking or gentle cycling.

- Finish with static stretches, focusing on major muscle groups like your legs, back, chest, shoulders, and arms.

- Hold each stretch for 15-30 seconds, focusing on breathing and relaxing into the stretch.

Remember, proper form and technique are essential for getting the most out of your workouts and preventing injuries. If you're new to exercise or unsure about any exercises, it's always a good idea to consult with a certified fitness professional who can guide you and provide personalized advice.

By following the Fit in Fifteen Workout Framework, you can ensure that your 15-minute workouts are effective, efficient, and enjoyable. Embrace the challenge, push yourself within your limits, and celebrate your progress along the way.

Chapter 5: Nutrition for Optimal Fitness (Trainer's Perspective)

Welcome to Chapter 5 of the "Fit in Fifteen Plan: Fitness for Busy People" eBook! As your personal trainer, I'm thrilled to dive into the world of nutrition and share practical insights to help you fuel your body for success. In this chapter, we'll explore the importance of balanced nutrition, energy balance, pre- and post-workout fueling, healthy snacking, hydration, mindful eating, and portion control. Let's embark on a journey to optimize your nutrition and enhance your fitness results!

The Importance of Balanced Nutrition: Proper nutrition is the cornerstone of your fitness journey. It's about nourishing your body with the right combination of macronutrients (carbohydrates, proteins, and fats) and micronutrients (vitamins and minerals). By incorporating a variety of nutrient-rich foods into your diet, you'll provide your body with the essential building blocks it needs for energy production, muscle repair, and overall well-being. For example, include complex carbohydrates like whole grains, lean proteins such as chicken breast or tofu, and healthy fats like avocado or nuts in your meals.

1. ## Energy Balance and Caloric Intake:
   Achieving an optimal energy balance is crucial for reaching your fitness goals. It involves balancing the calories you consume with the calories you burn through physical activity. To determine your daily caloric needs, consider factors such as your age, gender, weight, height, and activity level. Whether your objective is weight loss, maintenance, or muscle gain, tracking your calorie intake can help you stay on track. For example, if your goal is weight loss, aim for a slight calorie deficit by

consuming fewer calories than you burn.

2.   Pre-Workout Nutrition: Fueling your body before workouts is key to maximizing performance and sustaining energy levels. Aim to have a pre-workout meal or snack that combines carbohydrates for readily available energy and proteins for muscle support. Consider options like a banana with peanut butter or Greek yogurt with berries. Timing is also important; aim to eat about 1-2 hours before your workout to allow for digestion and absorption.

3.   Post-Workout Nutrition: After a challenging workout, your body needs proper nutrition to recover and repair. Focus on consuming a combination of carbohydrates and proteins within 30-60 minutes of completing your workout. This helps replenish glycogen stores and supports muscle protein synthesis. Examples of post-workout meals or snacks include a protein shake with fruit, a turkey wrap with whole wheat bread, or a grilled chicken salad with quinoa.

4.   Healthy Snacking and Meal Planning: Healthy snacking is an excellent way to maintain energy levels throughout the day. Opt for nutrient-dense snacks like carrot sticks with hummus, Greek yogurt with granola, or a handful of almonds. When it comes to meal planning, aim to prepare meals in advance to ensure you have nutritious options readily available, even on busy days. Cook larger portions of lean proteins, whole grains, and vegetables, and portion them into containers for easy grab-and-go meals.

5. **Hydration and Its Impact on Performance:** Staying hydrated is essential for optimal performance and overall health. Proper hydration helps regulate body temperature, supports digestion, and transports nutrients to your cells. Aim to drink water consistently throughout the day and increase your intake before, during, and after workouts. Carry a water bottle with you to stay hydrated on the go and listen to your body's thirst signals as a reminder to drink.

6. **Mindful Eating and Portion Control:** Mindful eating involves being present and aware of your eating habits, making conscious food choices, and practicing portion control. Slow down and savor each bite, paying attention to your body's hunger and full

Example Meals

1. Breakfast (15 minutes):

- Option 1: Smoothie Bowl: Blend together a mix of your favorite fruits, leafy greens, and a liquid of your choice (such as almond milk or coconut water). Pour the smoothie into a bowl and top with toppings like granola, nuts, or coconut flakes.

- Option 2: Yogurt Parfait: Layer Greek yogurt, sliced fruits, and a sprinkle of granola or nuts in a small glass or bowl.

- Option 3: Avocado Toast: Toast a slice of whole grain bread, spread mashed avocado on top, and add a sprinkle of salt and pepper. Optionally, you can add sliced tomatoes or a poached egg for extra flavor.

2. Lunch (15 minutes):

- Option 1: Protein Salad: Toss mixed greens with a lean protein source, such as grilled chicken, tofu, or chickpeas. Add a variety of chopped vegetables, like cucumbers, cherry tomatoes, and bell peppers. Drizzle with a light dressing of your choice.

- Option 2: Wrap or Roll-Up: Take a whole grain wrap or lettuce leaves and fill them with your choice of lean protein, veggies, and a spread like hummus or mustard. Roll it up and enjoy.

- Option 3: Quinoa Bowl: Cook quinoa according to package instructions and top it with cooked vegetables, a lean protein source, and a drizzle of dressing or sauce.

3. Dinner (15 minutes):

- Option 1: Stir-Fried Veggies and Tofu: Quickly sauté a mix of colorful vegetables and tofu in a pan with a splash of low-sodium soy sauce or other desired spices. Serve over a bed of brown rice or quinoa.

- Option 2: Shrimp or Fish Tacos: Sauté shrimp or fish in a pan with your preferred seasonings. Fill small tortillas with the cooked seafood, along with shredded cabbage, diced tomatoes, and a squeeze of lime juice.

- Option 3: One-Pot Vegetable Soup: Simmer a combination of vegetables, broth, and your choice of protein (such as diced chicken or beans) in a pot until cooked through. Season with herbs and spices for added flavor.

These meal options are designed to be smaller in portion size, yet packed with nutrients to fuel your body effectively. Remember to eat mindfully and take your time to enjoy each bite. If necessary, you can also portion out the meals in advance for even quicker consumption.

Additionally, consider incorporating healthy snacks like sliced fruits, raw vegetables, or a handful of nuts throughout the day to keep your energy levels stable and satisfy any cravings.

As always, be mindful of any dietary restrictions or allergies you may have and adjust the meal options accordingly. With these quick and nutritious meals, you can stay on track with your fitness goals even on the busiest of days. Let's make every minute count towards your health and well-being!

Chapter 6: Recovery and Self-Care (Trainer's Perspective)

Welcome to Chapter 6 of the "Fit in Fifteen Plan: Fitness for Busy People" eBook! In this chapter, we'll explore the importance of recovery and self-care in your fitness journey. As your personal trainer, I want to emphasize the significance of giving your body the rest and care it needs to optimize your results and overall well-being. Let's dive into some key principles and practices to help you enhance your recovery and prioritize self-care.

1. Understanding the Importance of Recovery:

- Rest and recovery play a crucial role in your fitness routine. Rest days allow your body to repair and rebuild muscle tissues, replenish energy stores, and reduce the risk of overuse injuries. Recognize the importance of listening to your body and providing it with the time it needs to recover.

2. Restorative Sleep:

- Quality sleep is essential for effective recovery and overall health. Aim for 7-9 hours of uninterrupted sleep each night. Establish a consistent bedtime routine, create a comfortable sleep environment, and minimize exposure to electronic devices before bed to promote better sleep.

3. Active Recovery:

- Engaging in active recovery activities can enhance blood flow, promote muscle repair, and reduce muscle soreness. Consider low-intensity exercises like walking, cycling, or swimming on rest days. These activities help increase circulation and facilitate recovery without putting excessive stress on your body.

4. Mobility and Flexibility:

- Incorporate regular mobility and flexibility exercises into your routine. Stretching and performing mobility exercises can improve joint range of motion, reduce muscle tension, and prevent injuries. Focus on areas that feel tight or are prone to stiffness, and dedicate a few minutes each day for these exercises.

5. Self-Care Strategies:

- Make self-care a priority in your routine. Engage in activities that help you relax, recharge, and rejuvenate. This can include taking a warm bath, prayer, reading a book, spending time in nature, or pursuing hobbies that bring you joy and fulfillment.

6. Proper Nutrition and Hydration:

- Proper nutrition and hydration are essential for recovery. Fuel your body with a balanced diet consisting of lean proteins, whole grains, fruits, vegetables, and healthy fats. Ensure you're drinking enough water throughout the day to support optimal hydration, as it plays a vital role in various bodily functions.

7. Stress Management:

- Chronic stress can negatively impact your progress and overall well-being. Find healthy ways to manage stress, engaging in activities you enjoy, seeking support from loved ones, or exploring stress management strategies that work best for you.

By prioritizing recovery and self-care, you'll create a sustainable and well-rounded fitness routine. Remember, taking care of yourself extends beyond physical exercise. Give yourself permission to rest, rejuvenate, and nurture your body and mind. Embrace the idea that recovery is an essential part of your fitness journey, and it will contribute to better results and long-term success.

As your trainer, I encourage you to implement these principles and practices into your routine. Strive for balance, listen to your body's needs, and give yourself the care you deserve. Together, we'll create a foundation for sustainable fitness and well-being. Let's make recovery and self-care a priority in your fitness journey!

Chapter 7: Staying Motivated and Overcoming Challenges (Trainer's Perspective)

Welcome to Chapter 7 of the "Fit in Fifteen Plan: Fitness for Busy People" eBook! In this chapter, we'll focus on staying motivated and overcoming challenges on your fitness journey. As your personal trainer, I understand that maintaining motivation and overcoming obstacles are key to achieving your goals. Let's explore strategies and techniques to help you stay motivated and conquer any challenges that come your way.

1. Setting Realistic Goals:

   - Begin by setting realistic and achievable goals that are specific, measurable, attainable, relevant, and time-bound (SMART goals). Break down your long-term goals into smaller milestones, making them easier to accomplish and track progress along the way.

2. Finding Your Why:

   - Dig deep and discover your underlying motivations for pursuing fitness. Understanding your "why" will give you a sense of purpose and drive during challenging times. It could be improving your health, boosting confidence, setting a positive example for loved ones, or simply wanting to feel better in your own skin.

3. Celebrating Milestones:

   - Celebrate your progress and accomplishments along the way. Acknowledge and reward yourself when you achieve a milestone or reach a goal. Treat yourself to something that aligns with your healthy lifestyle, such as a massage, new workout gear, or a fun fitness-related activity.

4. Tracking Your Progress:

- Keep a record of your workouts, measurements, and any other relevant data. Tracking your progress allows you to see how far you've come and provides motivation to keep pushing forward. Use a fitness journal, mobile app, or even a simple spreadsheet to monitor your achievements.

5. Variety and Fun:

- Incorporate variety into your workouts to keep things interesting and prevent boredom. Try new exercises, join fitness classes, or participate in outdoor activities. Finding activities that you genuinely enjoy will make your fitness routine more fun and sustainable in the long run.

6. Partnering Up:

- Find an exercise buddy or accountability partner to share your fitness journey with. Working out with someone else can provide motivation, support, and a sense of camaraderie. You can challenge and inspire each other, making the process more enjoyable and engaging.

7. Adapting to Challenges:

- Recognize that challenges are a natural part of any fitness journey. Rather than seeing them as setbacks, view them as opportunities for growth and learning. Adapt your approach when faced with obstacles, modify your workouts if necessary, and seek guidance from professionals if needed.

8. Positive Self-Talk:

- Develop a positive mindset and practice self-compassion. Be kind to yourself, especially during challenging times. Replace negative self-talk with affirmations and encouraging statements. Believe in your ability to overcome obstacles and remind yourself of the progress you've already made.

Remember, motivation is not constant, and it's normal to have ups and downs. It's essential to stay committed to your goals and implement strategies that keep you engaged and focused. With the right mindset and tools, you can overcome challenges and maintain your motivation throughout your fitness journey.

As your trainer, I'm here to support and guide you. Reach out for help when needed, stay consistent, and never lose sight of why you started. You have the power to overcome any challenge that comes your way. Let's stay motivated, stay committed, and make your fitness goals a reality!

Chapter 8: Sustaining Your Fitness Journey (Trainer's Perspective)

Welcome to Chapter 8 of the "Fit in Fifteen Plan: Fitness for Busy People" eBook! In this chapter, we'll focus on sustaining your fitness journey in the long term. As your personal trainer, I understand that creating lasting lifestyle changes is essential for achieving and maintaining your fitness goals. Let's explore strategies and techniques to help you sustain your progress and continue leading a healthy, active life.

1. Embracing a Growth Mindset:

- Adopt a growth mindset, which means believing in your ability to learn and improve over time. Understand that setbacks and challenges are part of the journey, and view them as opportunities for growth and self-improvement. Embrace a mindset of continuous learning and be open to new ideas and approaches.

2. Prioritizing Consistency:

- Consistency is key when it comes to sustaining your fitness journey. Make exercise and healthy habits a non-negotiable part of your routine. Set a schedule that works for you and stick to it as closely as possible. Even on busy days, aim for at least a few minutes of activity to keep the momentum going.

3. Building a Supportive Community:

- Surround yourself with a supportive community of like-minded individuals who share your fitness goals and values. Join fitness groups, participate in online communities, or find workout buddies who can provide encouragement, accountability, and motivation.

Having a support system can make a significant difference in staying motivated and engaged.

4. Continuously Setting New Goals:

- Keep your fitness journey exciting and challenging by continuously setting new goals. Once you achieve a milestone, set a new target to work towards. This will help you stay focused and motivated, as well as provide a sense of accomplishment as you reach each new goal.

5. Educating Yourself:

- Stay informed and educated about various aspects of fitness, nutrition, and overall wellness. Read books, follow reputable fitness blogs, attend workshops or seminars, and consult with professionals in the field. The more knowledge you acquire, the better equipped you'll be to make informed decisions and sustain your fitness journey.

6. Practicing Mindful Eating:

- Maintain a healthy relationship with food by practicing mindful eating. Pay attention to your body's hunger and fullness cues, choose whole, nutrient-dense foods, and savor each bite. Avoid restrictive diets or excessive calorie counting, and instead focus on nourishing your body with balanced and sustainable nutrition.

7. Incorporating Active Lifestyle Habits:

- Look for opportunities to incorporate physical activity into your daily life. Take the stairs instead of the elevator, walk or bike to nearby destinations, and find activities you enjoy that keep you moving. Cultivate an active lifestyle that extends beyond structured workouts, making physical activity a natural part of your day.

8. Staying Flexible and Adaptable:

   - Recognize that life is full of changes and unexpected circumstances. Be flexible and adaptable in your approach to fitness. If your schedule gets hectic, modify your workouts or find creative ways to stay active. Embrace adaptability and find solutions that work for you in different situations.

By implementing these strategies, you'll create a sustainable fitness journey that lasts a lifetime. Remember, it's not about quick fixes or temporary results but rather about making lasting changes that promote a healthy and active lifestyle.

As your trainer, I'm here to guide and support you on your journey. Embrace the process, stay committed to your goals, and keep pushing forward. Sustaining your fitness journey is possible, and with the right mindset and strategies, you'll continue to thrive and enjoy the benefits of a healthy lifestyle. Let's make your fitness journey a lifelong adventure!

Chapter 9: Incorporating Fitness into a Busy Lifestyle (Trainer's Perspective)

Welcome to Chapter 9 of the "Fit in Fifteen Plan: Fitness for Busy People" eBook! In this chapter, we'll explore strategies for incorporating fitness into a busy lifestyle. As your personal trainer, I understand the challenges of balancing work, family, and other responsibilities while prioritizing your health and fitness. Let's delve into practical tips and techniques to help you seamlessly integrate exercise and healthy habits into your busy schedule.

1. Time Management:

   - Start by assessing your schedule and identifying available time slots for exercise. Look for pockets of time throughout your day, such as early mornings, lunch breaks, or evenings. Prioritize your workouts by scheduling them as appointments in your calendar, treating them with the same importance as other commitments.

2. Efficient Workout Techniques:

   - Make the most of your limited time by incorporating high-intensity interval training (HIIT) and circuit training into your workouts. These techniques involve short bursts of intense exercise followed by brief recovery periods, maximizing calorie burn and overall fitness gains in a shorter time frame.

3. Multitasking Exercises:

   - Maximize your efficiency by incorporating multitasking exercises that work multiple muscle groups simultaneously. Examples include squats with overhead presses, lunges with bicep curls, or planks with leg raises. These compound exercises save time while delivering a full-body workout.

4. Active Transportation:

- Look for opportunities to incorporate physical activity into your daily commute or errands. Consider walking or biking instead of driving short distances, using stairs instead of elevators, or taking active breaks during your workday. These small changes add up and contribute to your overall fitness.

5. Prioritizing Non-Negotiable Fitness Time:

- Identify specific time slots that are non-negotiable for your fitness routine. Treat these slots as sacred and guard them against other distractions or obligations. Communicate your commitment to family, friends, and coworkers, so they understand and respect your dedicated fitness time.

6. Fitness Apps and Online Workouts:

- Take advantage of technology by using fitness apps or accessing online workout platforms. These resources offer a wide range of guided workouts that you can do at home or on the go, eliminating the need for a gym or travel time. Choose workouts that align with your preferences and time constraints.

7. Incorporating Active Breaks:

- Break up long periods of sitting or sedentary work by incorporating active breaks. Set a timer every hour to remind yourself to stand up, stretch, and move around for a few minutes. Consider walking meetings, using a standing desk, or doing quick exercises during your breaks to keep your energy levels up.

8. Preparing Healthy Meals in Advance:

- Plan and prepare your meals in advance to ensure you have nutritious options readily available, even on busy days. Batch cook and portion meals, pack healthy snacks, and have a supply of pre-cut fruits and vegetables. This saves time and helps you make healthier choices when time is limited.

9. Finding Accountability and Support:

- Seek accountability and support from others who share similar fitness goals. Join fitness groups, participate in online challenges, or find an accountability partner who can keep you motivated and on track. Engaging with a supportive community provides encouragement and helps you stay committed.

Remember, incorporating fitness into a busy lifestyle requires intentional planning and commitment. By implementing these strategies, you can make exercise and healthy habits a seamless part of your daily routine. Adapt them to fit your unique schedule and preferences, and be flexible when unexpected changes occur.

As your trainer, I'm here to guide and support you in finding the right balance. Embrace the mindset that every small step towards a healthier lifestyle matters. With dedication, consistency, and a bit of creativity.

Chapter 10: Maintaining Long-Term Success (Trainer's Perspective)

Welcome to Chapter 10, the final chapter of the "Fit in Fifteen Plan: Fitness for Busy People" eBook! In this chapter, we'll focus on maintaining long-term success in your fitness journey. As your personal trainer, I understand that sustaining the progress you've made and continuing to lead a healthy lifestyle requires ongoing commitment and dedication. Let's explore strategies and practices to help you maintain your achievements and enjoy lifelong success.

1. Embracing a Growth Mindset:

 - Adopt a growth mindset and view your fitness journey as a continuous process of growth and improvement. Be open to learning new things, trying different approaches, and adapting to changes. Embrace challenges as opportunities for personal development and use setbacks as lessons to propel you forward.

2. Regular Goal Setting:

 - Set new goals regularly to keep yourself motivated and engaged. Whether it's improving your strength, increasing endurance, or achieving a specific fitness milestone, having goals gives you something to strive for. Make sure your goals are realistic, measurable, and align with your overall vision of health and wellness.

3. Periodizing Your Training:

 - Implement a periodization plan in your training to prevent plateaus and maintain progress. Periodization involves dividing your training into specific phases, each with different focuses and intensities. This approach helps prevent burnout, promotes continued adaptation, and keeps your workouts fresh and exciting.

4. Continuing Education:

- Stay updated with the latest fitness trends, research, and techniques by continuing your education in the field. Attend workshops, seminars, or webinars, read books and articles, and engage with fitness professionals and experts. Continuously expanding your knowledge will enhance your understanding and improve your ability to sustain success.

5. Mindful Eating and Nutrition:

- Maintain a balanced and mindful approach to eating. Focus on nourishing your body with whole, nutrient-dense foods, and practice portion control. Be aware of emotional eating triggers and develop strategies to address them. Stay hydrated and listen to your body's hunger and fullness cues for optimal nutrition and energy.

6. Consistency and Routine:

- Stay consistent with your exercise routine and healthy habits. Make physical activity and self-care a priority in your daily life. Schedule your workouts and treat them as important appointments. Create a routine that works for you, ensuring that exercise and healthy choices become ingrained habits rather than occasional indulgences.

7. Regular Assessments and Adjustments:

- Periodically assess your progress and reassess your goals. Take measurements, track your performance, and evaluate your overall well-being. Based on the results, make necessary adjustments to your training, nutrition, or lifestyle. This continual self-assessment allows you to make informed decisions and maintain long-term success.

8. Self-Care and Recovery:

- Prioritize self-care and recovery as integral parts of your fitness journey. Get sufficient sleep, manage stress levels, and incorporate rest days into your training plan. Listen to your body and give it the time it needs to rest, repair, and rejuvenate. Remember that optimal health and performance require a balanced approach.

9. Accountability and Support:

- Surround yourself with a supportive community of like-minded individuals who share your commitment to health and fitness. Seek accountability partners, join fitness groups, or work with a coach or trainer who can provide guidance and support. Engaging with others who have similar goals will help you stay motivated and accountable.

10. Celebrate Milestones and Enjoy the Journey:

- Take time to celebrate your achievements and milestones along the way. Acknowledge the progress you've made and reward yourself with non-food-related treats that align with your healthy lifestyle. Embrace the journey, enjoy the process, and find joy in the daily practices.

Conclusion: Celebrating Your Achievements and Embracing a Lifelong Fitness Journey (Trainer's Perspective)

Congratulations on reaching the final chapter of the "Fit in Fifteen Plan: Fitness for Busy People" eBook! Throughout this journey, you've learned valuable strategies and techniques to help you lead a healthy, active life, even with a busy schedule. As your personal trainer, I'm immensely proud of your commitment and dedication to your fitness goals.

Remember that fitness is not just a destination; it's a lifelong journey. As you conclude this eBook, I want to emphasize the importance of celebrating your achievements and embracing the ongoing process of self-improvement. Here are some final thoughts to keep in mind as you continue your fitness journey:

1. Reflect on Your Progress:

Take a moment to reflect on how far you've come since you started this program. Celebrate the milestones you've achieved, whether it's an increase in strength, improved endurance, or better overall well-being. Recognize your dedication and the positive changes you've made in your life.

2. Embrace Consistency and Adaptability:

Maintaining your fitness journey requires consistency, but it also demands adaptability. Life is full of unexpected twists and turns, and your ability to adapt and adjust your approach will be crucial. Be flexible in your workouts, nutrition, and mindset, and find solutions that work for you in different situations.

3. Set New Goals:

Keep the momentum going by setting new goals that challenge and inspire you. Use the knowledge and skills you've gained from this program to continue growing and evolving. Whether it's conquering a new fitness milestone, trying a different workout style, or exploring a new aspect of wellness, keep pushing yourself to new heights.

4. Seek Support and Accountability:

Surround yourself with a supportive community that shares your passion for health and fitness. Seek out accountability partners, join fitness groups, or consider working with a coach or trainer who can guide and motivate you. Having a support system will help you stay on track and provide the encouragement you need during challenging times.

5. Embrace Balance and Enjoyment:

Remember that fitness is not just about hard work and discipline—it's about finding balance and enjoying the process. Find activities you genuinely enjoy and make them a regular part of your routine. Seek joy in the small victories, savor the progress you make, and allow yourself to find fulfillment in the journey itself.

6. Be Kind to Yourself:

Above all, be kind to yourself throughout your fitness journey. Celebrate your successes, but also embrace your imperfections and setbacks. Treat yourself with compassion and self-care, and remember that each day is an opportunity to start fresh and make choices that align with your goals and values.

As your trainer, I'm here to support you on your ongoing fitness journey. Remember that fitness is a lifelong endeavor, and the lessons you've learned during this program will continue to guide you. Stay committed, stay motivated, and never lose sight of the incredible potential within you.

Now, go out there and continue to thrive. Embrace a healthy, active lifestyle, and let your fitness journey be an inspiring example for others. Thank you for trusting me as your guide, and I wish you continued success and happiness in all your fitness endeavors. Keep up the amazing work!

Appendix

As a coach, I understand that continuing your fitness journey requires ongoing support and access to valuable resources. That's why I've included this comprehensive appendix filled with resources and tools to help you achieve sustained success in your fitness endeavors.

1. Recommended Fitness Apps and Websites:

   - Fitness Apps: MyFitnessPal, Nike Training Club, Fitbod, Seven - 7 Minute Workout

   - Fitness Websites: Bodybuilding.com, Fitness Blender, Darebee, Nerd Fitness

2. Fitness Equipment Recommendations:

   - Resistance Bands: Perform Better Exercise Bands, Fit Simplify Resistance Loop Bands

- Kettlebell: CAP Barbell Cast Iron Kettlebell, Yes4All Vinyl Coated Kettlebell

- Foam Roller: TriggerPoint GRID Foam Roller, LuxFit Premium High-Density Foam Roller

3. Sample Workout Plans:

- Full-Body HIIT Circuit: Combining bodyweight exercises like squats, push-ups, burpees, and planks into a high-intensity circuit.

- Strength Training Split: Dividing your workouts into different muscle groups, such as legs, chest and back, shoulders and arms, and core.

- Cardio Interval Training: Alternating between bursts of high-intensity exercises like sprints or jump rope and active recovery periods.

4. Nutrition and Recipe Resources:

- Nutrition Websites: ChooseMyPlate.gov, Academy of Nutrition and Dietetics, Nutrition.gov, Healthline

- Recipe Websites: Skinnytaste, EatingWell, Fit Men Cook, Deliciously Ella

5. Tracking and Progress Tools:

- Fitness Journals: Fitlosophy Fitbook, Clever Fox Fitness Planner

- Mobile Apps: MyFitnessPal, StrongLifts 5x5, Strava, Apple Health

- Wearable Devices: Fitbit, Garmin, Apple Watch, Whoop

6. Recommended Reading List:

- "Atomic Habits" by James Clear

- "The Power of Now" by Eckhart Tolle

- "Becoming a Supple Leopard" by Dr. Kelly Starrett

- "Mindset: The New Psychology of Success" by Carol S. Dweck

These examples provide a starting point, but feel free to explore other options and find what works best for you. Remember, these resources are meant to enhance your fitness journey and provide you with additional support and knowledge along the way.

Glossary: Key Terms and Definitions

To help you better understand the concepts and terminology used throughout the book, here is a glossary of key terms and their definitions:

1. High-Intensity Interval Training (HIIT): A training method that alternates between short bursts of intense exercise and brief periods of rest or low-intensity activity.

2. Cardiovascular Exercise: Physical activities that increase heart rate and promote cardiovascular fitness, such as running, cycling, swimming, or aerobics.

3. Resistance Training: A form of exercise that involves using external resistance, such as weights or resistance bands, to build strength, endurance, and muscle mass.

4. Bodyweight Exercises: Exercises that use your body weight as resistance, such as push-ups, squats, lunges, and planks, to improve strength and flexibility.

5. Repetitions (Reps): The number of times an exercise is performed in a set.

6. Sets: A group of repetitions performed consecutively without rest.

7. Rest Interval: The period of time between sets or exercises for recovery and regeneration.

8. Macronutrients: Essential nutrients required in large amounts by the body, including carbohydrates, proteins, and fats, which provide energy and support various bodily functions.

9. Micronutrients: Essential nutrients required in smaller amounts by the body, including vitamins and minerals, which play crucial roles in growth, development, and overall health.

10. Portion Control: The practice of eating appropriate portion sizes to manage caloric intake and maintain a balanced diet.

11. Mindful Eating: The practice of paying attention to the present moment and being fully aware of the eating experience, including the taste, texture, and satisfaction derived from food.

12. Body Composition: The proportion of fat, muscle, and other tissues in the body, often measured as a percentage of body fat.

13. Periodization: A systematic approach to training that divides the overall training program into distinct phases, each with specific goals, intensity levels, and exercises to optimize performance and prevent plateaus.

14. Recovery: The process of allowing the body to repair and adapt after exercise, involving rest, proper nutrition, and techniques like stretching or foam rolling.

15. Motivation: The internal or external factors that drive and sustain behavior, such as setting goals, finding enjoyment in exercise, or seeking support from others.

This glossary will help you navigate the terminology used in the book and deepen your understanding of key concepts. Refer to it whenever you come across unfamiliar terms to enhance your comprehension and make the most out of your fitness journey.

Acknowledgments

I would like to take this opportunity to express my gratitude to all those who have contributed to the creation and realization of this book. Their support, guidance, and encouragement have been invaluable in bringing this project to fruition.
And most of all I would like to thank my Lord and Saviour Jesus Christ for giving me his life in exchange for mine.

First and foremost, I would like to thank my family for their unwavering support throughout this journey. Your belief in me and constant encouragement have been a driving force behind my efforts. I am grateful for your love and understanding, which allowed me the time and space to dedicate myself to this project.

I extend my deepest appreciation to my editor and the publishing team at Jehu Press for their expertise and guidance. Your meticulous attention to detail and insightful feedback have played a significant role in shaping this book into its final form.

I would also like to acknowledge the countless individuals who have contributed their knowledge, expertise, and experiences to the fitness community. Your research, teachings, and passion for health and wellness have inspired me and countless others on our own fitness journeys.

Lastly, I want to express my gratitude to the readers of this book. Your decision to embark on a journey towards better health and fitness is commendable. I hope that the information, guidance, and insights provided within these pages empower you to make positive changes and achieve your fitness goals.

Remember, the path to fitness is not always easy, but it is worth every effort. Embrace the challenges, celebrate the victories, and never lose sight of the incredible potential within you.

Thank you all for your unwavering support and belief in this
project.
God Bless,

David B